D1567779

HILDEGARDE E. PEPLAU

Notes on Nursing Theories

SERIES EDITORS

Chris Metzger McQuiston
Doctoral Candidate, Wayne State University

Adele A. Webb
College of Nursing, University of Akron

Notes on Nursing Theories is a series of monographs designed to provide the reader with a concise description of conceptual frameworks and theories in nursing. Each monograph includes a biographical sketch of the theorist, origin of the theory, assumptions, concepts, propositions, examples for application to practice and research, a glossary of terms, and a bibliography of classic works, critiques, and research.

HILDEGARDE E. PEPLAU

Interpersonal Nursing Theory

Cheryl Forchuk

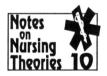

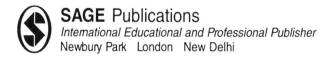

SAGE Publications
International Educational and Professional Publisher
Newbury Park   London   New Delhi

For information address:

SAGE publications, Inc.
2455 Teller Road
Newbury Park, California 91320

SAGE publications Ltd.
6 Bonhill Street
London EC2A 4PU
United Kingdom

SAGE Publications India Pvt. Ltd.
M-32 Market
Greater Kailash I
New Delhi 110 048 India

Printed in the United States of America

Library of Congress Cataloging-in-Publication Data

Forchuk, Cheryl.
    Hildegard E. Peplau: interpersonal nursing theory / Cheryl
Forchuk.
        p. cm.—(Notes on nursing theories; 10)
    Includes bibliographical references.
    ISBN 0-8039-4857-3 (cl). — ISBN 0-8039-4858-1 (pb)
    1. Nursing—Philosophy. 2. Nurse and patient. 3. Nursing—
Psychological aspects. 4. Peplau, Hildegard E.   I. Title.
II. Series: Notes on nursing theories; v. 10.
    [DNLM: 1. Peplau, Hildegard E. 2. Nursing Theory. 3. Nurses—
biography.   WY 86 F697h 1993]
RT84.5.F67 1993
610.73′01—dc20
DNLM/DLC   93-28310

93 94 95 96 10 9 8 7 6 5 4 3 2 1

Sage Production Editor: Diane S. Foster

163082

AAX-5690

Contents

Foreword

Theory has become a compelling interest within the nursing profession since the mid-20th century. Many nurses have been focusing on theory, defining what it is, and discussing how it is produced, how it is tested clinically and how it is generated by various nursing research methods. Since the 1950s several different theoretical frameworks have been published by nurses. These theories have spawned considerable discussions, comparisons, many conferences, publications, as well as major changes in nursing education curricula. Out of this ferment of ideas, a knowledge base called "nursing science" is evolving.

The knowledge that a profession uses in its work is the product of many scholars who research, refine, and build upon their own work as well as upon theories that their colleagues have published. This book is an illustrative example.

Dr. Cheryl Forchuk has devoted years of sustained study to the work that I have published. She has traced it to its roots, reviewed assessments of the work made by other scholars, and subjected the theoretical framework to critical analysis and to considerable research testing in clinical practice of psychiatric nursing. In this text, the substance of my published work is put forth in an updated, clearly organized form and in easily readable style. Dr. Forchuk has enriched the work by providing many illuminating examples of application in the current practice of nursing.

It is a distinct honor for me to have the remarkable intelligence and sustained effort of Dr. Forchuk brought to bear upon my work, originally published four decades ago. I am very proud to have been a minor participant in the creative reordering as presented in this publication.

This book portrays significant scholarship applied to a theoretical framework that has had a definitive impact upon the practice of nursing. It also suggests a model of the kind of careful scrutiny that is central to the knowledge building trend currently in process within the nursing profession.

HILDEGARD E. PEPLAU
Professor Emerita
Rutgers University

Acknowledgment

The ongoing assistance and support of Hildegard Peplau is gratefully acknowledged.

I would also like to acknowledge the loving support from my husband, Gerry Smits; my children, Ian, Robin, and Callista; and my mother, Dorothy Forchuk.

Biographical Sketch of the Nurse Theorist: Hildegard E. Peplau, BA, MA, Ed.D.

Born: Sept. 1, 1909
Position: Professor Emerita, Rutgers University, New
    Brunswick, NJ
Registered Nurse: Pottstown, Pennsylvania Hospital School of
    Nursing
BA: (interpersonal psychology) Bennington College,
    Bennington, VT
MA: (teaching and supervision of psychiatric nursing)
    Teachers' College, Columbia University, New York, NY
Ed.D: Teachers' College, Columbia University, New York, NY
Fellow: American Academy of Nursing
Other: Honorary Doctorates from University of Indianapolis,
    Rutgers University, Columbia University, Duke
    University, Boston College, and Alfred University; and
    numerous other honors.

1

Peplau's Theory: Origins

Introduction

Peplau stated that she began her theory development in response to "the need in the late 1940s to develop 'advanced psychiatric nursing' for graduate programs in psychiatric nursing. The available nursing literature in psychiatric nursing at that time was not in any way adequate for graduate level, university-based psychiatric nursing education programs" (personal correspondence, December 23, 1990). Her original intent was not theory development but "only to convey to the nursing profession ideas [she] thought were important to improve practice" (personal correspondence, July 1989).

Peplau's first book, *Interpersonal Relations in Nursing*, was published in 1952 (1952a, reissued in 1988 and 1991). This book outlined her conceptual framework for psychodynamic nursing. Peplau's conceptual framework signified the end of a long drought in the development of nursing theory; it was the first published nursing theory development since Nightingale.

Origins of the Theory

Dr. Peplau first studied interpersonal relations theory in the 1930s-1940s at Bennington College (personal correspondence, December 23, 1990). This interpersonal focus underpinned her later theory development.

Peplau, strongly influenced by the interpersonal development model of Harry Stack Sullivan (1952), incorporated his theory of personality development and the self system in her work. Peplau, like Sullivan, was also influenced by the early work of symbolic interactionists such as George Hubert Mead (1934). Examples of the influence of symbolic interactionism can be seen in the focus on social influences on personal development and with the idea that communication involves the use of symbols. Other influences include Rollo May's (1950) work on anxiety and the understanding of learning developed by Miller and Dollard (1941).

Peplau's 1952 work was grounded in interpersonal theory and the clinical experiences of herself and students. Peplau stated "concepts emerged from practice—my own and supervisory review of graduate student nurses beginning in 1948—from actual nurse-patient-relationship data" (personal correspondence, August 1989).

Since 1952, Peplau has been a prolific writer. She published a second book in 1964, dictated a series of 20 audiotapes to teach and communicate her theory, and has published more than 80 chapters and articles. Her work has endured over the years and is widely used in clinical practice. Sills (1978) reviewed several prominent nursing journals and found that references to Peplau's work had not only been sustained but actually had increased over the years.

Two recent Canadian surveys (Martin & Kirkpatrick, 1987, 1989) found that in a tertiary care psychiatric hospital, approximately two thirds of the nursing staff used Peplau's theory as a basis for their practice. Similarly, an American survey (Hirschmann, 1989) of mental health nurses in private practice found that approximately half were guided by Peplau's theory.

Although Peplau's theory has been most frequently used by psychiatric or mental health nurses, Peplau believed psychodynamic nursing transcended all clinical nursing specialties and that all nursing is based on the interpersonal process and relationship that develops between the nurse and client.

2

Peplau's Theory: Assumptions, Concepts and Propositions

Introduction

Assumptions are basic beliefs within a given theory that are accepted as true. One must accept the given assumptions of a theory in order to adopt it. The concepts are the major components or building blocks of the theory. Propositions describe the relations among concepts.

Assumptions of the Theory

In Peplau's 1952 book she identified two "guiding assumptions" that were underpinnings to her framework. These were:

1. The kind of nurse each person becomes makes a substantial difference in what each client will learn as she or he is nursed throughout her or his experience with illness (p. xi).
2. Fostering personality development in the direction of maturity is a function of nursing and nursing education; it requires the use of principles and methods that permit and guide the process of

grappling with everyday interpersonal problems or difficulties (p. xi).

Peplau (1989d; personal correspondence, December 1990) has also stated as assumptions that:

3. Nursing can take as its unique focus the reactions of clients to the circumstances of their illnesses or health problems (1989d, p. 28).

4. Since illness provides an opportunity for learning and growth, nursing can assist clients to gain intellectual and interpersonal competencies, beyond those that they have at the point of illness, by gearing nursing practices to evolving such competencies through nurse-client interactions (1989d, p. 28). Peplau references Gregg (1954) and Mereness (1966) in the development of this fourth assumption.

Additional implicit and explicit assumptions identified by Forchuk (1991c)[1] include:

5. Psychodynamic nursing crosses all specialty areas of nursing. It is not synonymous with psychiatric nursing since every nurse-client relationship is an interpersonal situation in which recurring difficulties of everyday life arise (summarized from Peplau, 1952a, introduction).

6. Difficulties in interpersonal relations recur in varying intensities throughout the life of everyone (Peplau, 1952a, p. xiv).

7. The need to harness energy that derives from tension and anxiety connected to felt needs to positive means for defining, understanding, and meeting productively the problem at hand is a universal need (Peplau, 1952a, p. 26).

8. All human behavior is purposeful and goal-seeking in terms of feelings of satisfaction and/or security (Peplau, 1952a, p. 86).

9. The interaction of nurse and client is fruitful when a method of communication that identifies and uses common meanings is at work in the situation (Peplau, 1952a, p. 284).

10. The meaning of behavior to the client is the only relevant basis on which nurses can determine needs to be met (Peplau, 1952a, p. 226).

11. Each person will behave, during any crisis, in a way that has worked in relation to crises faced in the past (Peplau, 1952a, p. 255).

Concepts of the Theory

Peplau's theory focuses on the interpersonal processes and therapeutic relationship that develops between the nurse and client. Figure 2.1 depicts the major concepts of Peplau's theory within this interpersonal perspective. The metaparadigm, or core concepts, of nursing includes: nursing, person, environment, and health. Peplau's theory defines the concepts of the metaparadigm in the following way:

1. *Nursing* is an educative instrument, a maturing force, that aims to promote health (Peplau, 1952a).
2. *Person* is an individual, developed through interpersonal relationships, that lives in an unstable environment (Peplau, 1952a).
3. *Environment* is physiological, psychological, and social fluidity that may be illness-maintaining or health-promoting (Peplau, 1952a, p. 82; 1973c; 1987a).
4. *Health* is forward movement of personality and other on-going human processes in the direction of creative and constructive personal and community living (Peplau, 1952a).

Interpersonal Focus

The interpersonal focus of Peplau's theory requires that the nurse attend to the interpersonal processes that occur between nurse and client. This is in sharp contrast to many nursing theories that focus on the client as the unit of attention. Although individual client factors are assessed, the nurse also self-reflects. The focus is the interpersonal process and relationships, not the constituent parts (or individuals). Interpersonal processes include: the nurse-client relationship, communication, pattern integration, and the roles of the nurse.

Nurse-Client Relationship

Peplau's interpersonal theory of nursing identifies the therapeutic nurse-client relationship as the crux of nursing. The nurse-client relationship evolves through identifiable, overlapping phases. The

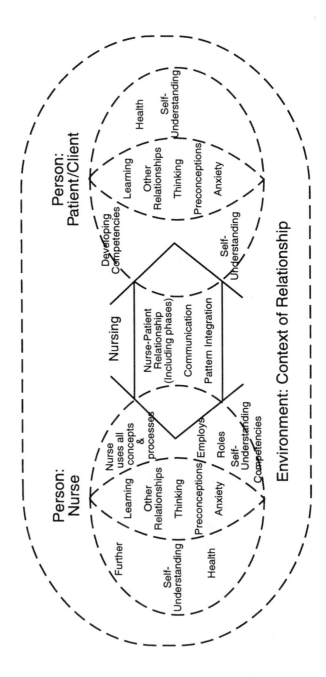

Figure 2.1. Peplau's Framework: Major Concepts and Their Interrelationships

8

phases include orientation, working, and resolution. The relationship form (see Figure 2.2), developed by Forchuk et al. (1986) and tested by Forchuk and Brown (1989), gives a pictorial overview of the nurse and client behaviors at each phase. The reliability and validity of the form was reported in Forchuk and Brown (1989).

The initial phase of the nurse-client relationship is the orientation phase where the nurse and client come to know each other as persons and the client begins to trust the nurse. The time in the orientation phase can vary from a few minutes of the initial meeting to months of regular sessions.

The second phase of the nurse-client relationship, the working phase, is subdivided into identification and exploitation subphases. In the identification subphase the client begins to identify problems to be worked on within the relationship. The nature of the problems identified can be as diverse as the scope of nursing practice. Examples include identifying inadequate pain management, requests for health teaching regarding breast feeding, or wanting to discuss unresolved issues related to past sexual abuse. The exploitation subphase occurs as the client makes use of the services of the nurse to work through the identified problems. Often, as initial problems are worked through, further problems are identified by the client.

The nurse does not "solve" the client's problems, but rather gives the client the opportunity to explore options and possibilities within the context of the relationship. For example, the nurse may provide information on community resources, or provide health teaching related to medication, illness, or health promotion if appropriate in the context of the relationship. However, the nurse employing Peplau's theory would resist all temptation related to "advice giving" because this would undermine the roles and responsibilities of the client.

The resolution phase of the relationship occurs between the time the actual problems are resolved and the relationship is terminated. Examples of work that may need to be done in this period include connecting the client to community resources, working through dependency issues in the relationship, learning preventative measures, strengthening social supports, and summarizing the work completed.

The nurse-client relationship does not evolve as a simple linear process. Although the relationship may be predominantly in one phase, reflections of all phases can be seen in each interaction. Every

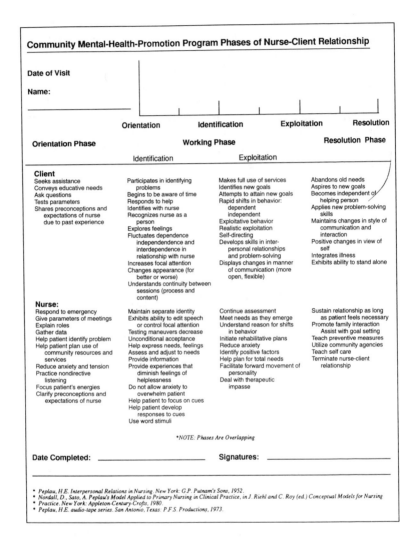

Figure 2.2. Relationship Form
SOURCE: Forchuk, C., & Brown, B. (1989, p. 32). Reprinted with permission.

interaction has a beginning (orientation), middle (working), and end
(resolution) that reflect the larger pattern of the ongoing nurse-client
relationship.

Communication

Communication includes both verbal communication and nonverbal communication. Verbal communication is expressed through language, while nonverbal communication is expressed through empathic linkages, gestures, postures, and patterns.

Verbal communication, or language, is important as a reflection of thought processes. This is obvious on the literal content level: For example, the client gives information on pain, on current abilities, or on perceptions of problems. However, in addition to the literal content, there are symbolic meanings, patterns, and underlying assumptions that can be conveyed through the choice of words or phrases. Consider the differences among the following statements: "I have a chronic migraine headache problem and it appears to be starting to flare up," "My head is killing me," and "I'm getting a headache." Different information is conveyed regarding ownership of the headache, possible intellectualizing, and degree of distress. However, one would not make immediate assumptions but rather be attentive to emerging patterns and validate these with the client (or better yet encourage the client to note the patterns and validate these with the nurse).

Peplau considers the use of verbal communication to be an essential component of the nurse-client relationship. She states, "The general principle is that anything clients act out with nurses will most probably not be talked about, and that which is not discussed cannot be understood" (1989a, p. 197). Talking about issues and concerns gives the client an alternative to acting out these issues.

Peplau (1973d) has described patterns of word usage that may require corrective action on the part of the nurse. Common patterns include:

1. Overgeneralization — For example, the client says, "The worst things always happen to me." The nurse would attempt to help the client be more specific by asking for one incident.
2. Inappropriate use of pronouns — A paranoid client may insist "they" are out to get him, and the nurse asks, "Who are they?"
3. The suggestion of automatic knowing through repetition of the phrase "you know" — The nurse conveys the information that "I only know what you tell me about it," and drops such phrases from his or her own language.

This corrective use of language is quite similar to approaches suggested by cognitive therapists such as Aaron Beck (1976) and Albert Ellis (1962). A difference is that cognitive therapy assumes one is directly changing the thought. Peplau believes one is changing the language, but because thought and language are part of an integral whole, a change in one is reflected in the other. Nonverbal language is more subtle than verbal language and may at times contradict the verbal message. Consider the example of the person who screams "I am not upset!" In such cases it is the nonverbal message that tends to be believed. Congruence is an important consideration for the nurse to monitor in his or her own communication. Empathy and caring can be transmitted on a nonverbal level, as can feelings such as indifference or hostility.

Most nonverbal communication is culturally influenced, so one must be cautious in transcultural interpretation and use of gestures. For example, does avoiding eye contact suggest dishonesty, shyness, or respect? It can depend on the cultural orientations of the sender and receiver of the message.

A personal example that exemplifies the need for awareness of cultural differences occurred in the author's work with a native Indian client. I had concerns about how the sessions were progressing. The client stated he felt things were going well. I could not identify what it was that was bothering me, but thought the problem might be culturally related. The client and I had one session videotaped to be viewed by a cultural anthropologist. The client and I viewed the videotape with the anthropologist and we all noticed the almost comical "dance of the eyes." He was attempting to avoid eye contact as I was attempting to maintain it. We discussed our different interpretations of eye contact (he avoided eye contact in deference to authority and out of respect, while I believed I was trying to maintain our open communication through eye contact). We agreed to not impose our rules on each other. However, the client noted that every time he went for a promotion interview, he was unsuccessful, and that the feedback I had given prior to the tape about "something not seeming quite right" was similar to the feedback he received after the interviews. He decided to use eye contact in job interview/promotion situations. Although I believe his success reflected more than a change in eye contact, that client was convinced that the two promotions he received in the next year were related to his new awareness of this difference in communication. This situation also exemplifies how learning in the nurse-client relationship can be used in other relationships, and that both nurse and client learn and grow in the therapeutic relationship.

Similar examples of nonverbal communications that can be interpreted very differently by different people include touching, hugging, smiling, passing flatulence, hand movements, comfortable social distances, crossing legs, gestures, offering food, and gift-giving. These can have vastly different cultural meanings to different groups and individuals. Therefore the nurse needs to be aware of issues related to differences in interpretation of nonverbal communication when providing care to a client from a different cultural group. The nurse, through self-reflection and clinical supervision, also needs to be aware of his or her own personal and cultural nonverbal patterns that might, at times, interfere with the evolving nurse-client relationship.

Pattern Integration

Each individual and each system have customary patterns of interacting with others. Pattern integrations are the products of the interaction of the patterns of more than one individual or system. Peplau (1973c; 1987a) has identified four common pattern integrations: complementary, mutual, antagonistic and mixed.

A *complementary* pattern integration involves patterns that are different yet fit together like parts of a jigsaw puzzle. The "fit" assists in ensuring the continuity of the single patterns that make up the integration. An example of this integration can be found with the nurse who insists on "helping" clients by doing things they could actually do for themselves. This could range from cutting their meat at dinner to arranging an out-patient appointment. A complementary pattern occurs when this nurse works with a dependent client who prefers that others make all possible decisions. The nurse and client will form a comfortable partnership that will make it difficult for either to change. A similar integration could be perpetuated on a larger systems level if this dyad worked in the context of a hospital that emphasized the accountability of the nurse but not the accountability or involvement in decision making of the client. Similar examples of complementary pattern integrations could include anger-withdrawal, domination-submission, and belittling others-belittling self.

A *mutual* pattern integration occurs when two or more interacting individuals/systems display a similar pattern. The multiple use of a single pattern also assists in the continuity of each similar pattern. A classic example from the nursing literature is the mutual-withdrawal pattern first identified by Gwen Tudor (1952/1970) as occurring between specific clients and staff on an in-patient psychiatric unit. Unfortunately, examples of this mutual pattern can still be found across nursing specialties: consider the placement of selected, less desirable, medical or surgical patients as far away from the nursing station as possible, or the early discharge of some community clients who give the impression they are not interested in interacting with the nurse, despite their ongoing personal health problems.

Additional examples of mutual pattern integrations include: mutual anger, mutual disrespect, and mutual self-denigration. Positive examples could include mutual respect or mutual concern. It is important to consider that the nurse should employ mutual pattern integrations only with those patterns that the nurse and client would want to perpetuate.

Antagonistic pattern integrations include the combination of different individual patterns that do not fit well together. The combination, therefore, creates a discomfort or disharmony that can be used as a motivation toward change. An example given by Peplau (1973c) is that of a client with an angry pattern with a nurse who is using an investigative approach ("Tell me about what's going on") rather than responding with a complementary (e.g., withdrawal) or mutual (e.g., also responding in anger) pattern. Obviously, this is the ideal integration for patterns that require change.

The antagonistic pattern can also occur at an individual or larger systems levels. An example of an antagonistic pattern at the larger systems level could occur with a client who feels most comfortable being dependent and letting others "take care" of him or her. An antagonistic pattern would emerge if this client was in a therapeutic environment that encouraged the participation and decision making of all individuals. It would become uncomfortable for the client to maintain dependent behaviors.

An even broader systems example of an antagonistic pattern would be the introduction of a nursing care delivery system that emphasizes the accountability of each nurse (e.g., primary nursing) into a traditional paternalistic hospital system. The traditional paternalistic system emphasizes centralized decision making rather than decision making and accountability at the staff level. Thus the nursing care delivery system would create an antagonistic pattern with the larger hospital system. If change is desired, it would be beneficial for the antagonistic pattern integration to occur as frequently as possible and at a variety of personal and larger systems levels.

Other examples of antagonistic pattern integrations include withdrawal-seeking out, dependance-promoting independence, and self-denigration-acceptance of self and others. It needs to be remembered that the inherent incongruence of antagonistic pattern integrations is anxiety producing. The resultant anxiety needs to be harnessed and channeled toward change. However, the anxiety also requires careful monitoring so that it does not become overwhelming. This issue is more fully discussed under the concept of anxiety.

Peplau (1987a) has also identified *mixed* or changing pattern integrations. These include a combination of the earlier identified pattern integrations. For example, a person may respond to another's anger by first getting angry himself/herself (reflecting a mutual pattern integration) and then withdrawing (reflecting a complementary pattern). Mutual-complementary combinations continue to reinforce individual patterns. Antagonistic pattern integration used in combination with a mutual or complementary integration will lose effectiveness in promoting change, since individuals are more likely to respond to patterns that reinforce familiar and comfortable personal patterns.

Roles of the Nurse

The nurse may enact several roles with the client. The roles depend on the needs of the client and the skills and creativity of the nurse. The possible roles will also be influenced by the nurse's position and agency policies. For example, a community nurse in a case management program may include a role related to cutting through red tape (the form filler role?) in order to ensure that appropriate services are in place for the client. A clinical nurse specialist may include roles that allow the nurse to transcend institutional or agency boundaries. Examples include following a client through different hospital and community settings. On the other hand, a staff nurse working a set shift may find more limitations to the type of roles he or she can offer to the client. The nurse needs to be aware of the possibilities and constraints so that accurate information can be conveyed to the client.

Peplau's (1952a) book includes the following examples of roles: stranger, resource person, teacher, leader, surrogate for significant others, counselor, arbitrator, change-agent, researcher, and technical expert. Regardless of other roles assumed, the nurse and client always begin the relationship as strangers to each other.

In her 1964 book, Peplau emphasized the importance of the counselor role and stated that this was the primary role to be undertaken by nurses in psychiatric-mental health nursing. Traditionally, psychiatric nurses had focused on surrogate roles, particularly parent surrogate roles, and the result was custodial care that minimized the potential for growth and change. Peplau (1964) stated: "If (nurses) are unable to contribute in a truly corrective manner to the care of mental patients, the traditional nurse-patient relationship will be usurped by those who can; and nurses will be shunted into the role of glorified custodian or superclerk" (p. 7).

The counselor role must be valued as the prime vehicle for the development of the nurse-client relationship. Frequently this involves individual counseling. Other modes, such as group work, community development, and family systems nursing are also appropriate. Within these modalities, the group, community, or family would be the "client" rather than the individual constituent members. As in the example of the individual as client, the nurse-client relationship would develop in phases, and the concepts of communication, both verbal and nonverbal, pattern integrations, and roles of the nurse would also be applicable.

Intrapersonal Processes

Although the primary focus within Peplau's theory is on *inter*personal processes, *intra*personal processes of both the client and nurse are also considered. Intrapersonal processes are processes that occur within the person, rather than between people. There is a strong interrelationship between interpersonal and intrapersonal phenomena: intrapersonal structures, processes, and changes develop through interpersonal activity. Examples of intrapersonal concepts within Peplau's theory include anxiety, learning, thinking, and competencies. Although each of these is observed on an individual level, these concepts have interpersonal implications.

Anxiety

Anxiety is an energy that emerges in response to a perceived threat. The threat could range from the physical to the metaphysical. Peplau (1989a) described the sequence of steps in the development of anxiety as including: holding expectations, expectations not met, discomfort felt, relief behaviors used, and relief behaviors justified (p. 281). The expectations can include things such as beliefs, needs, goals, wishes, and feelings. The relief behaviors also cover a wide range of possibilities: aggression, withdrawal, compulsive behavior, psychosomatic complaints, hallucinations, delusions, sexual activity, risk-taking behavior, denial, intellectualizing, drug use, humor, self-reflection, discussion with others, validation, and problem solving to seek the sources of difficulty. These are only a few of the relief behaviors that can be used.

People (not just clients) generally develop patterns of relief behaviors that they tend to use over and over again. Obviously, some of these patterns are more helpful than others. Anxiety is often a basis for the client to seek assistance from the nurse. At times, problems created through these relief behaviors bring the client to seek the services of the nurse. At other times the client seeks assistance because he or she finds the relief behaviors inadequate in relieving the anxiety.

Peplau (1989a) describes how the nurse can assist the client to channel anxiety productively. First, the client needs to be aware of and be able to name the anxiety. Then, the client needs to see the connection between the anxiety and the relief behavior. Finally, the client formulates and states expectations. This final part of the process includes an understanding of the connection between held expectations and what actually happened and consideration of factors amenable to control (p. 282). Working through this process usually takes place over time and during several interactions. The author has had some experiences with chronic mental health clients where it has taken months for the client to even be aware of and to name the anxiety.

Anxiety has been described by Peplau as existing along a continuum including mild, moderate, severe, and panic. Although it is possible to experience a state of no anxiety (euphoria), this seldom occurs. As human beings we constantly face a barrage of information and other stimuli that pose at least some minor threat to our self-views. Therefore, in most nurse-client encounters, both the nurse and client will be experiencing some anxiety.

As a person's anxiety increases, that person's focus of attention becomes increasingly narrow. At the lower end of the anxiety continuum, this may actually be useful in assisting the person to focus on important details. A common example would be writing an exam without being aware of other people or distractions in the room. However, at higher levels of anxiety, the focus of attention may become so narrow that the individual only sees small details without being able to see the larger picture. A similar example would be the student who becomes so concerned about one exam item that the total time is spent on that item and the exam is not completed. For similar reasons, problem solving may be enhanced at lower levels of anxiety but inhibited as anxiety increases. The nurse and client need to monitor anxiety levels and attempt to keep the levels at the mild to moderate levels.

Peplau (1973a) describes how the nursing approach must take into consideration the current anxiety level of the client. For example, as the client's anxiety is increased, the nurse would need to use increasingly short, concrete sentences in order to be understood. At the severe or panic levels, it would be inappropriate to use sentences with more than two or three words. It may be that even these short sentences will not be understood by the client in panic, and the nurse will need to use presence as a simple nonverbal communication. The nurse also needs to be aware of the impact of anxiety on the client's current problem-solving abilities and learning abilities and adjust accordingly. Generally at severe or panic levels of anxiety no new learning can take place.

Anxiety can be transmitted interpersonally (Peplau, 1989a). It is for this reason that the nurse needs to monitor his or her own anxiety. The anxious nurse will communicate the anxiety to the client and vice versa. A common situation where this can occur is when the client feels out of control and the nurse fears a physical threat. This situation can easily escalate to a self-fulfilling prophecy (i.e., the client loses control and becomes assaultive). Such situations can more easily be prevented by intervening with the anxiety at lower levels and not allowing one's own anxiety to escalate the situation.

Learning

Peplau has described eight stages in the learning process. These are: (a) to observe, (b) to describe, (c) to analyze, (d) to formulate, (e) to validate, (f) to test, (g) to integrate, and (h) to utilize (Peplau, 1971b). Each stage in the learning process is also a competency. Therefore, as one's learning increases so do one's competencies.

Different individuals will be at different competency levels within the stages of learning. Even within one individual a wide degree of variation is possible. For example, a person with generally high learning abilities may have a dramatic drop in such abilities when faced with a high anxiety-producing situation.

It is important that the nurse determine the current stage of learning of the client so that appropriate comments can be made to build on the current level and to assist the client to move to the next level. For example, if the client is at the very basic level of only being able to observe but unable to share the observations, the nurse would ask simple questions related to observation. Peplau (1971b) gives examples of basic questions as "What do you see?" and "What is that noise?" As the person responds to these questions, he or she begins movement to the next stage—to describe.

There is an assumption that all people will at least be able to observe on some level, even if they cannot respond. For example, even with a comatose client the nurse could use the assumption of the ability to observe. The nurse in this situation may say, "I am now going to wash your face," and recognize the client's ability for some level of observation.

Forchuk and Voorberg (1991), in a program evaluation of a community mental health program based on Peplau's theory, found that clients were able to increase their current stage of learning. For example, upon admission, 60% of the clients with chronic mental illnesses were at the first stage of learning. Only 20% remained at this level after 2 years.

Thinking: Preconceptions and Self-Understanding

Thinking is an internal cognitive process. The thoughts of another person can only be inferred through observation of language and behavior. The concept of thinking may be particularly important for the nurse working with clients experiencing difficulty with their thinking processes. Examples include clients with thought disorders related to chronic mental illnesses such as schizophrenia, clients with developmental handicaps, and clients with organic brain disorders or brain injuries. The section on communication describes the integral relationship between thought and language as well as appropriate approaches to assist clients with their thinking through the use of language.

Specific thinking processes of both the nurse and client will impact on the evolving nurse-client relationship. These include the preconceptions the nurse and client have of each other and the self-understanding of the nurse and client.

Preconceptions are the initial impressions the nurse and client have of each other, before they know each other. The preconceptions may be formed through stereotyping, gossip, or past experiences with persons considered to be similar to the partner in the new dyad. Forchuk (1992a) found both the nurses' and clients' preconceptions of each other were highly predictive of progress in the evolving therapeutic relationship. She also found that these initial impressions were quite stable, with very little change over the first 6 months of the relationship. This study underlined the importance of consideration of both nurse and client factors. The nurse needs to be aware of preconceptions of the client, particularly negative impressions that may impede progress in the relationship. Similarly, client impressions should also be explored. If negative preconceptions cannot be worked through, a therapeutic transfer of the client to another nurse should be considered.

Self-understanding is also a specific thinking pattern that may influence the evolving relationship. However, within Peplau's theory, the concept of self-understanding has an unequal importance for the nurse and client. Self-understanding is considered to be a critical attribute of the nurse. Through self-reflection and supervision, the nurse needs to be constantly aware of how her or his own issues and behaviors are influencing the relationship. It is expected that the nurse's self-understanding will grow through therapeutic work with clients.

Clients may also experience an increase in self-understanding through the therapeutic relationship. However, an increase in interpersonal and problem-solving competencies is the client-related goal of the relationship rather than self-understanding. Self-understanding is a helpful side effect of the process of developing these competencies.

Competencies

Competencies are skills that have evolved through practice. Peplau (1973b) states that we all have numerous interpersonal and problem-solving capacities, but in order to become competencies, these must be developed over time and through practice. The nurse-client relationship provides a venue for the development of capacities into competencies. For example, learning to share selected experiences verbally may be a capacity that the client has not developed; it may be developed during the time spent with the nurse. Other examples of competencies/capacities include sitting for 5 minutes in the presence of another person, discussing one topic for 5 minutes, learning to trust, describing one's feelings to another person, identifying personal goals, and choosing a strategy to move toward a specific goal. From these examples it can be seen that there are a wide variety of competencies and that which ones develop will vary considerably with different client situations. The specific competencies evolve through the developing relationship.

It is expected that the nurse will also develop competencies through the evolving relationship. These would also be primarily of a problem-solving or interpersonal nature. For example, the nurse may learn how a specific person copes with hallucinations, may learn to remain silent for longer periods of time to allow the client the opportunity to initiate conversation, or may develop increased empathy for a certain life situation. As the nurse's competencies grow, so does his or her ability to help other people in similar situations. However, it is the client's development of competencies, not the nurse's, that is the priority. Parallel to the nurse's development of self-understanding, the nurse's competencies develop as a beneficial side effect of the therapeutic relationship. The client's competencies develop as a goal of the therapeutic relationship.

Although the idea that the client's competencies take priority may seem obvious, it is sometimes forgotten in practice. It often appears more expedient for the nurse to complete an activity (e.g., feeding, making a bed, setting an out-patient appointment, listing alternatives, searching out community resources, summarizing progress) rather than the client. Of course, if this occurs, the nurse develops the competency rather than the client.

Clinical Phenomena

Peplau encourages nurses to be aware of patterns with clinical phenomena. Observing patterns in the development and resolution of specific clinical issues allows learning from one clinical situation to potentially assist in others. This in no way negates the uniqueness of each situation and each client. It recognizes that each person and situation, although unique, can reveal aspects of a larger pattern.

Examples of clinical concepts that Peplau has explored are loneliness and hallucinations. Concepts are defined and operationalized with the identification of critical attributes. This would include the observable behaviors associated with the clinical phenomena. For example, observable signs that a person is having auditory hallucinations might include talking to an unobserved person and describing hearing voices in one's head. The nurse could identify a client with such behavior as having a pattern consistent with auditory hallucinations. Such behaviors may also be consistent with other patterns, for example the pattern of a peak religious experience. In this section, the clinical concepts of loneliness and hallucinations are very briefly described as examples of clinical phenomena.

Loneliness

Peplau (1989c) describes the problem of loneliness. She defines this as "an unnoticed inability to do anything while alone" (p. 256). This is contrasted with lonesomeness (a wish to be with others) and aloneness (being without company). She describes the development of loneliness through difficult early interpersonal relationships.

Peplau (1989c) describes the importance of the nurse being aware of clients' defenses of loneliness; examples include time-oriented complaints (endless days), relating to others in an overly familiar or anonymous manner, planlessness, or overplanning.

The nurse assists the client with loneliness through the establishment of a therapeutic relationship, which will include contact and limit setting. Where appropriate, the nurse and client also plan for potentially positive peer relationships.

Hallucinations

Peplau (1989a) defines hallucinations as consisting of "illusory figures, perceived *as if* they were real" (p. 312). Peplau describes the phases through which hallucinations develop in an attempt to avoid anxiety and mitigate loneliness.

The nurse needs to be aware that the experience of hallucinations seems very real to the client. The nurse will carefully use language that does not reinforce the existence of the hallucinations as being a mutually experienced reality. For example, the nurse might say, "What do the voices you are hearing say?" Peplau (1989a) states that the client needs to learn alternative ways of coping with anxiety and loneliness so that the hallucinations are not needed (pp. 319-324).

In summary, Peplau has identified a wide range of concepts that impact on the practice of the nurse and the evolving nurse-client relationship. These include interpersonal factors, intrapersonal factors, and specific clinical phenomena.

Propositions

Relations between major concepts in Peplau's theory are summarized in Table 2.1, which was originally published in Forchuk (1991a). From Table 2.1 it can be seen that the concepts are all interrelated, and that a change in one concept generally is reflected by further changes of other concepts. Most critically, the evolving nurse-client relationship moves the client through growth and therefore health.

Notes

1. Reprinted with permission of Chestnut House Publications. Copyright 1991.

TABLE 1.1 Concepts and Relations

	NURSING is related to:	PERSON is related to:	HEALTH is related to:	ENVIRONMENT is related to:	INTERPERSONAL RELATIONSHIPS (I.P.R.s) are related to:
PERSON	Nursing is a process between persons (nurse and patient).				
HEALTH	Health is the goal of nursing.	Health is within the person.			
ENVIRONMENT	Environment provides the context of nursing.	The person is within the environment.	Health is within the person, who in turn is within the environment. The environment can be health promoting or illness maintaining.		
INTERPERSONAL RELATIONSHIPS (I.P.R.s)	I.P.R.s are the crux or essential processes of nursing (critical attribute).	I.P.R.s are participated in by persons.	I.P.R.s contribute to a person's health (antecedent) and a person's health will in turn influence ongoing I.P.R.s (consequence).	The environment forms the context of I.P.R.s (critical attribute).	
COMMUNICATION	Communication occurs in nursing (critical attribute).	Communication occurs between persons.	Communication facilitates health, by contributing to I.P.R.'s (intervening).	Communication occurs within the context of the environment, and is part of the environment.	Communication occurs within interpersonal relationships (critical attribute).
PATTERN INTEGRATION	Pattern integrations occur in nursing (critical attribute).	Pattern integration occurs between persons.	Pattern integrations can facilitate health, by contributing to ongoing I.P.R.s (intervening).	Pattern integrations are a part of the environment (critical attribute).	Pattern integrations occur within Interpersonal relationships (critical attribute).

ROLES	Roles are the means for conducting nursing.	Roles are used by the nurse to promote health within the patient.	Roles are used by the nurse to promote health.	Roles are used in the context of the environment.	Roles are used within Interpersonal relationships (critical attribute).
THINKING	Thinking occurs in nursing as a prerequisite and critical attribute.	Thinking occurs within persons (critical attribute).	Self-understanding can promote health. Preconceptions can impede or promote health depending on their impact on interpersonal relationships (intervening).	Thinking is a within-person phenomenon occuring in context of the person within the environment.	Self-understanding can promote I.P.R.s. Preconceptions can promote or hinder I.P.R.s and vice versa.
LEARNING	Learning occurs in nursing as a consequent.	Learning occurs within persons (critical attribute).	Learning promotes health.	Learning is a within-person phenomenon occuring in the context of the person within the environment.	Learning occurs within the context of I.P.R.s. The interactions between learning and I.P.R.s can enhance or hinder each other.
COMPETENCIES	Competencies develop as a consequence of nursing (intermediate to promoting health).	Competencies develop within persons.	The development of competencies promotes health.	Competencies are a within-person phenomenon occuring in the context of the person within the environment.	Competencies occur within the context of I.P.R.s and can assist in the development of I.P.R.s.
ANXIETY	Anxiety occurs in nursing (critical attribute).	Anxiety occurs within and between persons (critical attribute).	Anxiety impedes health at severe or panic levels.	Anxiety is a within-person phenomenon occuring in the context of the person within the environment.	Anxiety impedes the developmet of relationships at severe or panic levels.

(Continued)

TABLE 1.1 (Continued)

	COMMUNICATION is related to:	PATTERN INTEGRATION is related to:	ROLES are related to:	THINKING is related to:	LEARNING is related to:	COMPETENCIES are related to:
PERSON						
HEALTH						
ENVIRONMENT						
INTERPERSONAL RELATIONSHIPS (I.P.R.s)						
COMMUNICATION						
PATTERN INTEGRATION	Pattern Integration and communication occur together in interpersonal relationships.					
ROLES	Roles require communication (prerequisite).	Roles are used by the nurse as part of the pattern integration.				

THINKING	Thinking is mediated through symbols (language). Changes in verbal communication reflect changes in thinking and vice versa.	Thinking occurs within the person and therefore indirectly interacts with pattern integration.	Thinking is required by the nurse in the selection and maintenance of appropriate roles.			
LEARNING	Communication promotes learning, and learning can then promote future communication.	Learning occurs within the person and therefore indirectly interacts with pattern integration.	Learning occurs with successful implementation of nurse roles, particularly the counselor and teacher roles.	Thinking is a prerequisite for learning, and learning, in turn, assists thinking.		
COMPETENCIES	Communication promotes the development of competencies.	Competencies occur within the person and therefore indirectly interact with pattern integration.	Competencies are developed through successful implementation of nurse roles, particularly the couselor and teacher roles.	Competencies are both a prerequesite for thinking, and further developed through thinking.	Competencies are learned by developing skills and capacities.	
ANXIETY	Anxiety impedes communication at severe or panic levels.	Anxiety occurs in the person and therefore indirectly interacts with pattern integration.	Anxiety at severe or panic levels will limit the appropriate roles to be used.	Anxiety impedes thinking when at severe or panic levels.	Anxiety impedes thinking when at severe or panic levels.	Anxiety at severe or panic levels impedes the development of competencies.

SOURCE: Forchuk, C. (1991c). Peplau's theory: Concepts and their relations. *Nursing Science Quarterly* 4(2) 54-60. Reprinted with permission.

3

---

*Application to
Practice and Research*

Introduction

$\times$ Peplau's theory can be used to guide both practice and research. Surveys of psychiatric nurses in both Canada (Martin & Kirkpatrick 1987, 1989) and the United States (Hirschmann, 1989) found at least half of the sample used Peplau's theory as a basis for practice. As well, Peplau's theory has been the basis of both quantitative research (for example, Forchuk, 1992a, 1992b) and qualitative research (e.g., Choiniere, 1991; Forchuk, et al., in progress).

Peplau's Theory in Practice

Peplau's theory can be used to guide the nurse in the various aspects of practice. It will be reflected in the focus of the assessment, the planned strategies, and the criteria used to evaluate the nursing care.

Assessment includes attention to the various concepts of the theory. The nurse would therefore focus on the interpersonal process of the relationship. A key consideration would be determining the current phase of the relationship. The nurse would employ various roles and be aware of communication and pattern integrations, particularly those occurring at the nurse-client level and the client-system level. The nurse would use self-reflection and self-awareness as well as observing and understanding phenomena related to the client. The nurse would be aware of the client's current level of learning. This awareness would assist the nurse to give comments and ask questions that can be appropriately understood and used to facilitate growth. The anxiety of both client and self would be monitored and approaches modified in context of the current levels of anxiety.

As an example, consider the situation the author encountered in working with Mrs. Oksana Fivechuk (a pseudonym). Mrs. Fivechuk was a 66-year-old inpatient in a long-term-care facility. She had not responded to a series of medications and treatments over the years. She had a long history of admissions for problems related to schizophrenia. Generally, as soon as her involuntary certificates expired, she would discharge herself against medical advice and refuse all aftercare. Admissions were generally precipitated by acute episodes where she would become extremely paranoid and refuse all medication, food, and drink. Staff were extremely frustrated and felt they were unable to help Mrs. Fivechuk out of this revolving door.

Preconceptions were very important to work through in the initial phase of the relationship. Mrs. Fivechuk had initiated conversation with the nurse because she identified by the nurse's name that they belonged to the same ethnic group. The nurse recognized this as an unusual opportunity because Mrs. Fivechuk generally avoided any interaction with staff.

An early question from Mrs. Fivechuk was, "Is your family from the Ukraine, or is that just your husband's name?" What it meant to be from the same ethnic group, and the numerous assumptions this entailed, were explored early in the relationship.

Mrs. Fivechuk's extreme paranoia was interwoven with her experience of having fled the Ukraine under difficult circumstances. She believed Russian spies were pursuing her, and during periods where her psychosis worsened, she believed almost everyone was entangled in plots to murder her. An example of an early assumption was that the nurse would have experienced similar persecution. This was not the case.

Testing was used extensively by the client for the initial 4 months. Examples included trying to extend the agreed-upon time for the duration of the interactions, or using the interactions to discuss other people's problems, dropping Russian phrases into the conversation to see if they were understood, and asking the nurse to figure out mathematical questions before allowing medications to be dispensed. Testing was understood as a strategy to establish if the nurse was a trustworthy person. Mrs. Fivechuk gradually accepted that it was appropriate to confide in someone with experiences different from her own.

The nurse also needed to be aware of preconceptions. Examples in this situation included cultural background, age (over 65), gender, diagnosis (schizophrenia), concern about the previous hospitalization pattern, and similarity to previous clients.

A language pattern used by Mrs. Fivechuk was vague use of pronouns. In particular, she would use the pronoun "they." At times this pronoun would be used in a normally socially acceptable manner. The phrase "you know" was peppered throughout her speech. An example of both is, "Well, you know what they say about people who eat too much." The nurse was aware that such phrases could reflect underlying difficulties with thinking patterns and would use questions like, "Who are you referring to when you say that?" or, "No, I don't know. Tell me about that." Exploring this particular statement with Mrs. Fivechuk allowed her to describe not eating as a means of avoiding potential poisoning. Later, after numerous questions related to "they," she was able to be more specific about people she did not trust rather than generalizing.

The process and experience of being able to trust another person is essential for the person suffering from paranoia. The nurse helped Mrs. Fivechuk use this trusting relationship to extend acceptance to other staff. Mrs. Fivechuk did not want to participate in group activities on the unit, but she did gradually begin to socialize with two other women on the ward. Gradually the circle of people that could be trusted grew larger. As Mrs. Fivechuk improved, a community nurse visited Mrs. Fivechuk on the ward so that the relationship could be established well before discharge. Mrs. Fivechuk became an active participant in the decision making related to her care and discharge into the community.

To determine the effectiveness of the nursing care provided, the nurse was aware of the passage through various stages of the therapeutic relationship. Critical client indicators included movement toward goals set by the client, including being able to confide with another person and being able to stay out of hospital for a longer period of time. Other client indicators were the ability to trust some others and remaining in hospital long enough for some therapeutic work to be accomplished, as well as physically recovering from the lack of food prior to admission. Further client progress was indicated through establishing a separate therapeutic relationship with the community nurse. Both the inpatient and community nurses also experienced growth through examining assumptions about the client.

The developing phases can also be seen in group work. A team of nurses worked with a group of clients with chronic mental health problems through a "ward community group" that focused on day-to-day issues. The clients had a minimum of 2 years' hospitalization with a diagnosis of chronic schizophrenia. Initially there was a lot of testing of parameters, for example, coming to the group late, coming and leaving, and disruptive behaviors such as singing or shouting. Clients initially raised relatively safe subjects and the staff involved tried to act very quickly on suggestions regarding the ward milieu. For example, there was concern expressed about the pay phone being just outside the ward rather than on the ward. The phone company was contacted and the phone moved.

Gradually the focus shifted from "What can the staff do?" to "What can we be doing together?" This paralleled the entry into the identification subphase of the working phase of the relationship. During this period clients organized several activities and cooperative ventures, such as a "coffee club." The coffee club involved pooling money, purchasing jars of coffee and related items, and organizing coffee times. This was cheaper than other coffee sources and had no direct staff input.

Clients identified that one aspect of their life that was very institutional was the way each day was similar to the the next. They contrasted this with a "normal" situation where the weekend is a time for rest. Continental breakfasts were organized for weekends so that clients could sleep in and have a less institutionalized lifestyle (i.e., weekends off). Staff arranged for communal supplies to be sent rather than individual meal trays, but the clients organized the activity and tidied up after themselves. The shift of activities from staff to clients was indicative of the exploitation phase of the relationship.

At regularly arranged periods, sessions of this ward community group were completed. Clients used this opportunity to review progress and also to evaluate directly the usefulness of the activity and make recommendations for future groups. Examples of recommendations included more groups per session and having clients participate in keeping minutes. The minutes were then read at the end of the group and beginning of the next group. This process and the end of each session reflected the resolution phase.

The phases of the relationship are useful for understanding group process. The staff participating in these groups would also use other aspects of Peplau's theory. They would attend to the anxiety level of the group and the language used. They would be aware of communication, both verbal and nonverbal, and of pattern integrations occurring on the personal and system levels. Changing from a common ward pattern of "helper-helpless" to a more collaborative style has been a difficult and ongoing process.

Peplau's theory has also been used to organize clinical programs. An example is the Community Mental Health Promotion Program of the Hamilton-Wentworth Department of Health Services (public health) in Hamilton, Ontario, Canada. This public health program offers case management services and counseling to individuals with a chronic mental illness who require service in their home. Staff found principles of Peplau's theory to be consistent with case management principles. This public health program is described in more detail in Forchuk et al. (1989).

The Relationship Form, outlining the phases of the relationship, is a part of the clinical record of the public health program. Similarly, a form based on Peplau's stages of learning is found on the chart. Only problems or issues agreed to by the client appear on the nursing care plan. The nurses use Peplau's theory as a guide to their practice. The program objectives (e.g., that clients will progress in therapeutic relationships) are drawn from the theory.

A formal evaluation consistent with Peplau's theory was used to evaluate the effectiveness of the overall public health program. Over a 2-year period, clients in the program were able to reduce hospitalization, develop therapeutic relationships, decrease social isolation, increase skills in activities of daily living, and increase their current stage of learning (Forchuk & Voorberg, 1991).

The Menninger Hospital in Topeka, Kansas, has adopted Peplau's theory as a basis for nursing care. The theory has been used despite a great variety in clientele, focus, and length of stay on various inpatient units.

The clinical examples given (except for the Menninger example) are drawn from the author's clinical experience and therefore reflect a psychiatric-mental health focus. This is not to suggest that this clinical specialty is the only appropriate venue for applying Peplau's theory. The importance of nurse-client relationships and related concepts transcends clinical specialty areas.

The nurse working in an emergency department who uses Peplau's theory will recognize that relationships there are frequently in the orientation phase and that clients are generally experiencing high levels of anxiety. This anxiety will affect the current learning phase. The nurse will therefore give clear parameters and will often use very short, simple sentences.

The nurse who uses Peplau's theory while working in a geriatric unit will be aware of the importance of establishing and maintaining a therapeutic relationship. That nurse may also find it particularly important to attend to language patterns as evidence of cognitive processes. The nurse observes pattern integrations, particularly family patterns, and attempts to promote ongoing healthy patterns.

The public health nurse using Peplau's theory may find the concept of stages of learning particularly useful in health teaching situations. The nurse is aware of the interrelationship between anxiety and learning. The nurse will at times work with clients who experience high levels of anxiety. Examples could include an inexperienced mother on a well-baby visit or a person receiving a disturbing diagnosis. The nurse adjusts the level of content appropriately and attends to the anxiety rather than focusing only on prepared content.

The nurse-manager guided by Peplau's theory would be aware of the importance of the nurse-client relationships. Such a nurse-manager will plan the organization of services so that consistent nurse-client assignment takes place. Every client will have a specific nurse assigned every shift and every effort will be made to maintain continuity of nurse-client assignments. When a client needs to undergo an anxiety-producing situation, for example chemotherapy or an unpleasant diagnostic test, the nurse-manager arranges for the regularly assigned nurse to accompany the client. The nurse-manager is aware of the importance of the fit between the nurse and client and would not promote the old adage, "a nurse is a nurse is a nurse." The nurse-manager would also find the concept of pattern integrations particularly useful in examining patterns of care and interaction from a broader systems perspective.

The nurse-educator using Peplau's theory would be aware of how his or her relationship with students parallels the stages of therapeutic relationships. This is well described in Buchanan (1993). The nurse-educator would also be aware of current stages of learning and how these could be affected by anxiety levels. Communication, both verbal and nonverbal, would be viewed as an essential vehicle for the learning process. The nurse-educator would realize that capacities become competencies through practice. He or she would therefore plan activities that encourage the practice of problem-solving and other skills.

Peplau's theory is most commonly used in psychiatric mental health nursing. However, these examples illustrate that the clinical utility of the theory extends beyond this nursing specialty.

Research

Research based on Peplau's theory should consider both nurse and client factors. Ideally such research should address the interpersonal factors and not just the intrapersonal factors of each participant in the relationship. Study of Peplau's theory can be done through quantitative and qualitative research designs. In this section, some of the past research involving Peplau's theory will be reviewed. In addition, the author's program of research focusing on the orientation phase of the nurse-client relationship will be described.

Peplau initially used a method similar to grounded theory in the development of her theory. In her 1952 book she advocated the use of process recordings or "nursing process forms" to study the nurse-client relationship (Peplau, 1952a, p. 308). Process recordings generally use a column format to record verbal and nonverbal communication of the nurse and client as well as nurse interpretations.

Early studies based on Peplau's work tended to use such process recordings. These were frequently published as case studies. Manaser and Werner (1964) published a collection of instruments that could be used in analyzing process recordings in a manner consistent with Peplau's framework.

Several examples of single case studies can be found in Burd and Marshall (1971) and Hays and Larson (1963). Examples of extensive case studies using process recordings include Hays and Myers (1964), who analyzed 106 hours of nurse-client interactions with respect to the levels of learning described by Peplau (1971b), and Lemmer (1988), who analyzed a series of 17 nurse-client interactions. A disadvantage of this approach is that it has usually been limited to the study of a single nurse-client dyad at a time, and generally no comparisons between dyads have been made. An exception is Thompson (1986), who compared two women receiving short-term individual therapy based on Peplau's theory.

Lego (1980) reviewed nursing literature published on the nurse-client relationship from 1946 to 1976. The vast majority of these publications involved single case studies and "of 166 clinical papers, 78 were written by students and faculty colleagues of Peplau" (p. 81).

A number of nurse-researchers have explored aspects of Peplau's theory through qualitative research methods. Morrison and Shealy (1992) have studied roles and role actions of the psychiatric nurse in the nurse-client relationship. This qualitative study included 30 registered nurses in 62 audiotaped interactions with children, adolescents, or adults who were psychiatric inpatients. Content analysis was conducted with respect to the roles undertaken by the nurses. The results were consistent with Peplau's (1964) contention that the counselor role was the primary role of the psychiatric nurse. There was a great deal of overlap among other common roles identified by Peplau, particularly leader and surrogate, and resource person and teacher. A secondary role of friend was identified. This role was one that was discouraged by Peplau (1952a). The context of the caregiving situation and client acuity were seen as influences in the roles assumed by the nurses.

Buchanan (in progress) is studying nurse-client relationships from the perspective of a group of nurses who have completed a certificate program in mental health nursing. The nursing program includes teaching Peplau's theory. This grounded theory study involves interviewing the nurses no sooner than one year following their completion of the program. Peplau's theory is used as a guiding framework for the development of collaborative helping relationships as part of the structural component of the clinical experience of the certificate program. Buchanan is particularly interested in the practicalities of attempting to use a specific theory in the work setting.

Initial analysis is consistent with Peplau's (1952a, 1988b) conceptualization of the phases of the nurse-client relationship. The practicalities of the work situation appear to influence the specific roles undertaken by the nurse. A discrepancy with Peplau's theory is that nurses tend to use self-disclosure more readily than Peplau's theory would recommend. This is very similar to the Morrison and Shealy (1992) finding regarding nurses' assuming a friend role with their clients.

Choiniere (1991) used a qualitative design to explore the development of trust between nurses and community mental health clients. Grounded theory was used to explore six clients' perceptions of nurse behaviors that facilitated the development of trust. This study found that trust was slow to evolve and took as long as 3 years to develop. The development of trust occurred through interlocking, overlapping phases (caring presence, interactive caring, and mutual caring) that were synchronous with the phases of the nurse-client relationship described by Peplau (1952a, 1988b).

Choiniere (1991) described trust as a learned end product of the exploitation subphase. Clients described a process that paralleled Peplau's stages of learning. Participants referred to *observed* patterns of the nurse that would be consistent with a trustworthy person. These patterns were then *described*, for example, as genuine concern and support. Participants *analyzed* the nurses' behaviors while *formulating* the belief that the nurses were trustworthy. This perception would be *validated* with the nurses, *tested, integrated,* and *utilized.*

The participants described the trust developed in the nurse-client relationship as having an effect beyond the dyad. Choiniere (1991) describes how clients stated that if their nurse believed them to be worthwhile persons, then perhaps they were. For example, one client stated that if her nurse could accept her as a worthwhile human being, then she could accept herself (p. 105).

The Relationship Form was developed by Forchuk and others (1986) to measure the phases of the nurse-client relationship as described by Peplau. It is a 7-point scale including the 4 phases of the relationship and 3 intermediate points. Forchuk and Brown (1989) have reported on the initial reliability and validity of the instrument. Peplau reviewed the Relationship Form for content validity. In addition, a panel of three independent clinical nurse specialists (CNSs), who functioned from an extensive theory-based practice, reviewed the instrument. Inter-rater reliability was established by having an additional CNS act as a blind rater by reviewing clinical records and comparing the phase to that determined on the form by the clinician in the nurse-client relationship. Agreement within 1 point of the 7-point scale was 91%, but crude diagonal agreement was only 41%. A problem noted was that, in cases where disagreement existed, the CNS consistently rated the relationship 1 point higher than the clinician.

To counterbalance the clinicians' hesitancy to note a change in the relationship until it has persisted for several encounters, a secondary confirmation was used in later studies by Forchuk and colleagues (Forchuk, 1992a; Forchuk et al., in progress). For example, the assigned nurse would validate the current phase with a blind (to other measures) clinical nurse specialist who practices from Peplau's framework (Forchuk, 1992a).

Forchuk and colleagues (Forchuk, 1992a, 1992b; Forchuk et al., in progress) have conducted several studies examining the orientation phase of the nurse-client relationship. This phase has been given particular focus because progress through this initial phase has been related to psychotherapy and rehabilitation outcomes (Gehrs, 1991; Kirtner & Cartwright, 1958; Saltzman, Leutgert, Roth, Creaser, & Howard, 1976).

Forchuk (1992b) reported on a study examining client demographic factors and their relation to the duration of the orientation phase. The 73 subjects were community clients of a mental health program. All clients had been diagnosed as having a chronic mental illness. This study was interesting in what was found *not* to be related to the duration of the orientation phase. Psychiatric diagnosis, age of client, gender of client, age of first psychiatric hospitalization, age of first psychiatric contact, and type of service received (long-term case management or problem-specific counseling) were all unrelated to the time in the orientation phase.

The only demographic factors that were related to the orientation phase were the number and length of psychiatric hospitalizations. Those clients who took 11 or more months in orientation also tended to take much longer for each psychiatric hospitalization (average 70.3 months hospitalization over 5.7 hospitalizations) when compared to the group who completed orientation in 2 or less months (averaged 10.9 months hospitalization over 4.1 admissions). A suggestion made in this study is that it is possible that information that would facilitate movement through the orientation phase would also facilitate shorter hospital admissions.

Forchuk (1992b) also examined situations where the client returned to the orientation phase after completing this phase. Through a record review, 30 cases where this occurred were identified. The context of the return to the orientation phase is revealing. In 17 of the cases, the return to the orientation phase accompanied a change in staff. It is interesting to note that some of these staff changes were very brief, for example, for vacation coverage. Where staff changes occurred it seemed important that the client be informed well ahead of time. In cases where clients had only 2 weeks' notice of a staff permanently leaving the agency, the clients took longer to work through the orientation phase with the new nurse than with the initial nurse. On the other hand, when the clients knew months in advance (with an obviously impending maternity leave), all clients were able to enter the working phase with the new nurse within 2 months.

The other 13 cases of clients' returning to the orientation phase accompanied a worsening of symptoms such as paranoia or depression. All of these clients returned to the working phase within 2 months, even if their symptoms persisted. Those clients with lengthier psychiatric hospitalizations appeared to be more likely to return to the orientation phase.

Forchuk (1992a) tested Peplau's theory regarding influences during the orientation phase. This investigation used a prospective design to examine the orientation phase of the nurse-client relationship. One hundred twenty-four newly formed nurse-client dyads constituted the sample. Client subjects were individuals with a chronic mental illness.

The following variables predicted by Peplau's theory to be related to development of the therapeutic nurse-client relationship were examined: (a) nurses' preconceptions of their clients, (b) clients' preconceptions of their nurses, (c) other interpersonal relationships of clients, (d) other interpersonal relationships of nurses, (e) anxiety of clients, and (f) anxiety of nurses. Variables were measured for both nurses and clients at 0, 3, and 6 months into their relationship.

Instruments used were the Relationship Form (Forchuk & Brown, 1989) to measure the duration of the orientation phase, the Working Alliance Inventory (Horvath & Greenberg, 1986) to measure the quality of the relationship, selected semantic differential scales

(Osgood, Suci & Tannenbaum, 1957) to measure preconceptions, Personal Resource Questionnaire (Brandt & Weinert, 1981; Weinert, 1987) to measure other interpersonal relationships, and the Beck Anxiety Scale (Beck, Epstein, Brown & Steer, 1988).

The preconceptions of both nurses and clients were most predictive of the developing relationship. Preconceptions of both nurses and clients were related to the duration of the orientation phase and development of the therapeutic alliance. There was support for the importance of clients' other interpersonal relationships but not nurses' other interpersonal relationships. Anxiety was not found to be significantly related to the development of the therapeutic relationship. A regression analysis including both nurse and client variables identified in the hypotheses was also completed. The explanatory power resulting from including both nurse and client variables was .38 ($R =$ .62). This is considerably greater than client factors alone ($R^2 = .17$, $R = .42$,), or the nurse factors alone ($R^2 = .14$, $R = .37$) as predictors of weeks in orientation.

This study therefore supported some tenets of Peplau's theory but not others. The finding that the combination of both nurse and client variables was most significant is supportive of an interpersonal approach. Many nursing theories focus on the client as the unit of attention, although the importance of the contribution of the nurse and larger social systems may be acknowledged. Peplau's theory recognizes that the nurse must use awareness of self and self-reflection as vigilantly as assessment of the client situation. This was reflected through the significance of the nurses' preconceptions.

A qualitative study examining the orientation phase of the relationship is currently being conducted (Forchuk et al., in progress). This naturalistic qualitative design will employ an interpersonal method drawing on the works of Peplau (1952a, 1988b) and ethnonursing (Leininger, 1985a; 1987; 1990). This study also involves clients with a chronic mental illness.

Nurses and clients are being interviewed during the orientation phase to explore their thoughts and feelings regarding the emerging relationship. Each interview will be conducted by a clinical nurse specialist who is also one of the principal investigators. The interviews will be unstructured and employ broad, open-ended questions related to the evolving nurse-client relationship. No predetermined questions will be used. The Relationship Form (Forchuk & Brown, 1989) is used to determine whether or not the dyad is still in orientation. Participants will be encouraged to talk about issues related to the nurse-client relationship. These interviews are being audiotaped. Nurse-client interactions are being videotaped during the orientation phase. Videotapes have been found particularly useful in identifying nonverbal issues. All audiotapes and videotapes are transcribed verbatim using Leininger's software program for qualitative data (Leininger, Templin, & Thompson, in progress). The qualitative study will involve the assistance of two well-known nursing theorists. Because the investigators have been primarily involved in work related to Peplau's theory (Forchuk, 1990, 1991a, 1991b, 1991c, 1992a, 1992b; Forchuk & Brown, 1989; Forchuk et al., 1989; Forchuk & Voorberg, 1991, Martin & Forchuk, 1989; Martin, Forchuk, Santopinto, & Butcher, 1992), it might be questionable how unbiased identification of themes might be. However, this investigation will be using validation with the study participants and a different theorist, Dr. M. M. Leininger (1985b, 1988). Using a different theorist avoids what Smith (1990) refers to as an "ideological circle." The circle can develop when the research method is based on a specific theory and the researchers are already committed to that theory. After the themes have been identified, a comparison will be made to the concepts and themes within Peplau's theory. Dr. Peplau has agreed to assist with this phase of the analysis. The investigators could not find an example of another nursing study employing two nurse theorists in any similar manner.

The primary aim of the qualitative investigation (Forchuk et al., in progress) is to identify clients' and nurses' perceptions of important influences in the nurse-client relationship during the orientation phase. A secondary purpose is to determine how the clients' and nurses' perspectives regarding the orientation phase of the therapeutic relationship relate to the theoretical framework proposed by Peplau (1952a). It is anticipated that the findings will assist nurses and clients in the establishment of therapeutic relationships.

The earlier quantitative study by Forchuk (1992a) and the ongoing qualitative study (Forchuk et al., in progress) will complement each other from both theoretical and methodological perspectives. The next step in the research program phase will include a meta-analysis of these two different studies. Future plans also include work with different clinical populations.

The examples of research using Peplau's theory reflect direct application to practice despite a broad diversity of methods used. Both qualitative and quantitative methods can be used in exploring issues from the perspective of Peplau's theory.

A key feature of such research is the inclusion of nurses and clients and the interpersonal focus.

Summary

Peplau's interpersonal theory of nursing identified the therapeutic nurse-client relationship as the crux of nursing. Her theory has been used extensively in nursing practice, particularly in mental health and psychiatric nursing. Peplau's theory allowed nursing to move away from "doing to" to "doing with" clients.

Glossary

Adaptation
A process employed to cope with the inevitable dilemmas of living. Synonyms include *adjust, fit,* and *conform* (Peplau, 1989a, p. 286).

Anxiety
An energy triggered by a perceived threat to the person's security. The threat could be real or imagined, internal or external. Levels of anxiety range from mild anxiety to moderate anxiety to severe anxiety to panic. Anxiety is considered a universally experienced phenomenon (Peplau 1952a, 1971a, 1973a, 1989a).

Behavior
Includes thoughts, actions, feelings and patterns (Peplau, 1989b, p. 201).

Capacities
Potential abilities that have not yet been developed.

Client
The recipient of nursing services. The client could be an individual, couple, family, group, or community (Forchuk, 1991c; Peplau, 1952b, 1987a, 1988a). Synonymous with *patient*.

Competencies
Skills or abilities that have evolved through the use and practice of capacities. Competencies evolving in the nurse-client relationship

include problem-solving and interpersonal competencies (Peplau, 1973b).

Communication
An interpersonal process to transmit information (ideas, feelings, attitudes) that includes verbal language and nonverbal communication (Peplau 1952a, pp. 289-307).

Environment
Physiological, psychological, and social fluidity that may be illness-maintaining or health-promoting (Peplau, 1952a, 1973c, 1987b).

Exploitation subphase
The second subphase of the working phase of the nurse-client relationship. This phase exists when the client is able to make full use of the services of the nurse and plans are put into operation (Peplau, 1952a, 1973g).

Goal of nursing
Forward movement of the personality (health) (Peplau, 1952a).

Health
Forward movement of personality and other ongoing human processes in the direction of creative, constructive, personal, and community living (Peplau, 1952a).

Identification subphase
The first part of the working phase of the nurse-client relationship. The client identifies with the nurse and the nurse-client encounters and begins to identify problems to be worked on within the nurse-client relationship (Peplau, 1952a, 1973g).

Illness maintenance
Pattern integrations that encourage the continued use of behaviors associated with the person's illness (Peplau, 1973c).

Interpersonal
Phenomena that occur between persons.

Interpersonal paradigm
The view that the therapeutic nurse-client relationship is the crux of nursing. This paradigm includes theorists such as Peplau, Orlando, Mellows, and Travelbee (Forchuk, 1991a).

Interpersonal relationships
Any processes occurring between two or more persons. Peplau includes Sullivan's (1952) perspective in specifying that all but one of the persons involved may be illusory (Forchuk, 1991c; Peplau, 1952a).

Intrapersonal
Phenomena that occur within the individual.

Investigative counseling
"An interviewing process that helps a person investigate life experiences" (Peplau, 1989b, p. 205).

Language
Verbal communication to express thoughts or feelings through words, images, concepts, or symbols. Peplau views thought and language as integral to each other (Peplau, 1973d).

Learning
Skill development generally acquired through an active interpersonal process. Stages of learning are: (a) to observe, (b) to describe, (c) to analyze, (d) to formulate, (e) to validate, (f) to test, (g) to integrate, and (h) to utilize (Peplau, 1971b).

Nonverbal communication
Any form of information exchange between two or more people that is not dependent on the use of language. These forms include empathic linkages, gestural or body messages, and patterns (Peplau, 1987a, pp. 203-204).

Nurse
The medium of the art of nursing. "The unique blend of ideals, values, integrity, and commitment to the well-being of others, expressed in a nurse's self-presentation and responses to clients, makes each nurse a one-of-a-kind artist in nursing practice" (Peplau, 1988a, p. 10).

Nurse-client relationship
The specific interpersonal relationship that develops between a nurse and a client. The relationship develops through interlocking and overlapping phases. These are: the orientation phase, the working phase (subdivided into identification and exploitation), and the resolution phase (Peplau, 1952a, 1962, 1964, 1965).

Nursing
An educative instrument, a maturing force, that aims to promote
health (Peplau, 1952a).

Orientation phase
The initial phase of the nurse-client relationship. The nurse and
client work through preconceptions, establish and meet parameters,
develop initial trust, and begin to understand each other's roles
(Peplau, 1952a, 1973e).

Panic
Extreme anxiety.

Patient
See Client.

Pattern integrations
Occur when the patterns of one person or system interact with
the patterns of another person or system. The pattern integrations
include complementary, mutual, antagonistic, and alternating. Pattern integrations may occur at several levels including intrapersonal, interpersonal, and systems phenomena (Peplau 1973c, 1987a,
1988a).

Patterns
A characteristic mode of behavior, a configuration of separate acts
or variations that have a similar aim or intention (Peplau, 1987a,
p. 204).

Person
An individual, developed through interpersonal relationships, that
lives in an unstable environment (Forchuk, 1991c; Peplau, 1952a).

Phases of the nurse-client relationship
Orientation, working (subdivided into identification and exploitation) and resolution (Peplau, 1952a, 1962; 1964; 1965).

Preconceptions
The initial thoughts, feelings and assumptions one person has about
another (Peplau, 1952a, pp. 21-30, 123).

Relief behaviors
Behaviors used to diminish or cope with anxiety (Peplau, 1989a).

Resolution phase
The final phase of the nurse-client relationship. It exists when all plans have been implemented until the nurse and client mutually agree to terminate the relationship (Peplau, 1952a, 1973f).

Roles of the nurse
The interlocking functions a nurse may undertake to assist a client (Forchuk, 1991e). Peplau (1952a) has identified common roles of the nurse as stranger, technical expert, surrogate for another person such as a parent or authority figure, teacher, resource person, and counselor. She further states that specific roles are variable within each nurse-client situation and are limited only by the imagination and skill of the nurse (Peplau, 1952a, pp. 43-72).

Self system
A person's concept of self that "is a product of socialization, a function in humans that evolves and is revised along constructive or destructive lines during interpersonal relationships throughout life" (Peplau, 1989a, p. 299).

Self-understanding
The extent to which a person has insight into his or her interpersonal and intrapersonal functioning. The self-understanding of the nurse will determine the extent to which the nurse can come to understand the situation confronting the client, from the client's perspective (Forchuk, 1991c; Peplau 1952a, foreword).

Theory
"A formulation of the meaning of observed phenomena in an order or form that enables the formulation to be used to explain similar phenomena . . . and to guide the professional in choosing interventions relevant to the phenomena observed" (Peplau, 1989d, p. 27).

Thinking
A process, mediated by language, by which experience is incorporated, stored, organized and recalled. Thinking is used to link experiences and for learning (Peplau, 1973d).

Working phase
The middle phase of the nurse-client relationship comprised of the identification and exploitation subphases. Problems are identified and worked through in this phase (Peplau, 1973g).

References

Beck, A. (1976). *Cognitive therapy and the emotional disorders.* Madison, CT: International Universities Press.

Beck, A., Epstein, N., Brown, G., & Steer, R. (1988). An inventory for measuring clinical anxiety: Psychometric properties. *Journal of Clinical and Consulting Psychology, 56,* 893-897.

Brandt, P. A., & Weinert, C. (1981). PRQ - A social support measure. *Nursing Research, 30*(5), 277-280.

Buchanan, J. (in progress). *A grounded theory study of the nurse-client relationship.* Unpublished manuscript, The University of New Brunswick, St. John, New Brunswick, Canada.

Buchanan, J. (1993). The teacher-student relationship: The heart of nursing education. In M. Rather (Ed.), *Transforming RN education: Dialogue and debate* (pp. 304-323). New York: NLN Publications.

Burd, S. F., & Marshall, M. A. (Eds.). (1971). *Some clinical approaches to psychiatric nursing.* London: Macmillan.

Choiniere, J. (1991). *Clients' perceptions of nurse behaviors that facilitate trust in nurse-client relationships.* Unpublished master's thesis, Saint Joseph College, West Hartford, CT.

Ellis, A. (1962). *Reason and emotion in psychotherapy.* Secaucus, NJ: Citadel Press.

Forchuk, C. (1989). *Peplau's framework: Concepts and their inter-relationships.* Unpublished manuscript, Hamilton Psychiatric Hospital, Hamilton, Ontario, Canada.

Forchuk, C. (1990). Peplau's interpersonal theory. In A. Baumann, N. Johnson, & D. Atai-Otaong (Eds.), *Decision making in psychiatric and psychosocial nursing* (pp. 22-23). Toronto: B. C. Decker.

Forchuk, C. (1991a). A comparison of the works of Peplau and Orlando. *Archives of Psychiatric Nursing, 5*(1), 38-45.

50   HILDEGARD E. PEPLAU

Forchuk, C. (1991b). Conceptualizing the environment of the individual with a
chronic mental illness. *Issues in Mental Health Nursing, 12,* 159-170.
Forchuk, C. (1991c). Peplau's theory: Concepts and their relations. *Nursing Sci-
ence Quarterly, 4*(2), 54-60.
Forchuk, C. (1992a). *The orientation phase of the nurse-client relationship: Testing
Peplau's theory.* Unpublished doctoral dissertation, Wayne State University,
Detroit, MI.
Forchuk, C. (1992b). The orientation phase: How long does it take? *Perspectives
in Psychiatric Care, 28*(4), 7-10.
Forchuk, C., Beaton, S., Crawford, L., Ide, L., Voorberg, N., & Bethune, J. (1986,
August). *A marriage between Peplau's theory and case management: Instrument
development.* Paper presented at the 1986 Nursing Theories Congress, Ryer-
son College, Toronto, Ontario, Canada.
Forchuk, C., Beaton, S., Crawford, L., Ide, L., Voorberg, N., & Bethune, J. (1989).
Incorporating Peplau's theory and case management. *Journal of Psychosocial
Nursing, 27*(2), 35-38.
Forchuk, C., & Brown, B. (1989). Establishing a nurse-client relationship. *Journal
of Psychosocial Nursing, 27*(2), 30-34.
Forchuk, C., & Voorberg, N. (1991). Evaluating a community mental health
program. *Canadian Journal of Nursing Administration, 4*(6) 16-20.
Forchuk, C., Westwell, J., Martin, M. L., Bamber, W., Kosterewa-Tolman, D., &
Hux, M. (in progress). *The orientation phase of the nurse-client relationship:
Exploration with an interpersonal method.* Unpublished manuscript, Hamil-
ton Psychiatric Hospital, Hamilton, Ontario, Canada.
Gehrs, M. (1991). *The relationship between the working alliance and rehabilitation
outcomes of clients with schizophrenia.* Unpublished master's thesis, Univer-
sity of Toronto, Ontario, Canada.
Gregg, D. (1954). The psychiatric nurse's role. *American Journal of Nursing, 54*(7),
848-851.
Hays, J., & Larson, K. (1963). *Interacting with patients.* New York: Macmillan.
Hays, J., & Myers, J. (1964). Learning in the nurse-patient relationship. *Perspec-
tives in Psychiatric Care, 2,* 20.
Hirschmann, M. J. (1989). Psychiatric and mental health nurses' beliefs about
therapeutic paradox. *Journal of Child Psychiatric Nursing, 2,*(1), 7-13.
Horvath, A. O., & Greenberg, L. (1986). The development of the Working Alliance
Inventory. In L. Greenberg & W. Pinsof (Eds.), *Psychotherapeutic process
handbook: A research handbook* (pp. 529-544). New York: Guilford.
Kirtner, W. L., & Cartwright, D. S. (1958). Success and failure in client-centered
therapy as a function of initial in-therapy behavior. *Journal of Consulting
Psychology, 22*(5), 329-333.
Lego, S. (1980). The one-to-one nurse-patient relationship. *Perspectives in Psychi-
atric Care, 18,* 67-89.
Leininger, M. M. (1985a). Ethnography and ethnonursing: Models and modes of
qualitative data analysis. In M. M. Leininger (Ed.), *Qualitative research methods in nursing* (pp. 33-72). Orlando, FL: Grune & Stratton.
Leininger, M. M. (1985b). Transcultural care diversity and universality: A theory
of nursing. *Nursing and Health Care, 6*(4), 209-212.

Leininger, M. M. (1987). Importance and use of ethnomethods: Ethnography and ethnonursing methods. In M. Cahoon (Ed.), *Recent advances in nursing* (pp. 12-15). London: Churchill Livingstone of Edinburgh.

Leininger, M. M. (1988). Leininger's theory of nursing: Cultural care diversity and universality. *Nursing Science Quarterly, 1*(4), 152-160.

Leininger, M. M. (1990). Ethnomethods: The philosophic and epistemic bases to explicate transcultural nursing knowledge. *Journal of Transcultural Nursing, 1*(2), 40-51.

Leininger, M. M., Templin, F., & Thompson, F. (in progress). *Leininger, Templin and Thompson program for qualitative analysis.* Detroit, MI: Wayne State University.

Lemmer, B. (1988). Care plan for a man receiving domiciliary care, using Peplau's model of nursing. In B. Collister (Ed.), *Psychiatric nursing: Person to person* (pp. 25-37). London: Edward Arnold.

Manaser, J. C., & Werner, A. M. (1964). *Instruments for the study of nurse-patient interaction.* New York: Macmillan.

Martin, M. L., & Forchuk, C. (1989, September). *Peplau's Theory: Application of theory-based practice.* Paper presented at the First National Clinical Nurse Specialists Conference, Hamilton, Ontario, Canada.

Martin, M. L., Forchuk, C., Santopinto, M., & Butcher, H. (1992). Alternative approaches to nursing practice: Application of Peplau, Rogers, and Parse. *Nursing Science Quarterly, 5*(8), 80-85.

Martin, M. L., & Kirkpatrick, H. (1987). *Nursing theories used by staff nurses.* Unpublished manuscript, Hamilton Psychiatric Hospital, Hamilton, Ontario, Canada.

Martin, M. L., & Kirkpatrick, H. (1989). *Nursing theories used by staff nurses: Two year re-evaluation.* Unpublished manuscript, Hamilton Psychiatric Hospital, Hamilton, Ontario, Canada.

May, R. (1950). *The meaning of anxiety.* New York: Ronald Press.

Mead, G. H. (1934). *Mind, self and society.* Chicago: University of Chicago Press.

Mereness, D. (1966). *Psychiatric nursing* (Vols. 1 & 2). Dubuque, IA: Brown.

Miller, N. E., & Dollard, J. (1941). *Social learning and imitation.* New Haven, CT: Yale University Press.

Morrison, E. G., & Shealy, A. H. (1992, September). *Work roles of the psychiatric staff nurse.* Paper presented at the 14th Southeastern Conference of Clinical Specialists in Psychiatric-Mental Health Nursing, Lexington, KY.

Osgood, C. E., Suci, G. J., & Tannenbaum, P. H. (1957). *Measurement of meaning.* Urbana: University of Illinois Press.

Peplau, H. E. (1952a). *Interpersonal relations in nursing.* New York: J. P. Putnam.

Peplau, H. E. (l952b). Psychiatric nurses family groups. *American Journal of Nursing, 52,* 1475-1477.

Peplau, H. E. (1962). Interpersonal techniques: The crux of psychiatric nursing. *American Journal of Nursing, 62,* 50-54.

Peplau, H. E. (1964). *Basic principals of patient counselling.* Philadelphia: Smith, Kline and French Laboratories.

Peplau, H. E. (1965). The heart of nursing: Interpersonal relations. *Canadian Nurse, 61,* 273.

Peplau, H. E. (1971a). Anxiety. In S. F. Burd & M. A. Marshall (Eds.), *Some clinical approaches to psychiatric nursing* (pp. 323-327). London: Macmillan.

Peplau, H. E. (1971b). Process and concept of learning. In S. F. Burd & M. A. Marshall (Eds.), *Some clinical approaches to psychiatric nursing* (pp. 333-336). London: Macmillan.

Peplau, H. E. (Speaker). (1973a). *Anxiety* (audio tape). San Antonio, TX: P. S. F. Productions.

Peplau, H. E. (Speaker). (1973b). *The concept of psychotherapy* (audio tape). San Antonio, TX: P. S. F. Productions.

Peplau, H. E. (Speaker). (1973c). *Illness maintaining systems* (audio tape). San Antonio, TX: P. S. F. Productions.

Peplau, H. E. (Speaker). (1973d). *Language and its relation to thought disorders* (audio tape). San Antonio, TX: P. S. F. Productions.

Peplau, H. E. (Speaker). (1973e). *The orientation phase* (audio tape). San Antonio, TX: P. S. F. Productions.

Peplau, H. E. (Speaker). (1973f). *The resolution phase* (audio tape). San Antonio, TX: P. S. F. Productions.

Peplau, H. E. (Speaker). (1973g). *The working phase.* (audio tape) San Antonio, TX: P. S. F. Productions.

Peplau, H. E. (1987a). Interpersonal constructs for nursing practice. *Nurse Education Today, 7*(5), 201-208.

Peplau, H. E. (1987b). Nursing science: A historical perspective. In R. Parse (Ed.), *Nursing science: Major paradigms, theories, and critiques* (pp. 13-30). Toronto: W. B. Saunders.

Peplau, H. E. (1988a). The art and science of nursing: Similarities, differences and relations. *Nursing Science Quarterly, 1*, 8-15.

Peplau, H. E. (1988b/1952). *Interpersonal relations in nursing.* London: Macmillan. (reissued)

Peplau, H. E. (1989a). Anxiety, self and hallucinations. In A. W. O'Toole & S. R. Welt (Eds.), *Interpersonal theory in nursing practice: Selected works of Hildegard E. Peplau* (pp. 270-326). New York: Springer.

Peplau, H. E. (1989b). Investigative counseling. In A. W. O'Toole & S. R. Welt (Eds.), *Interpersonal theory in nursing practice: Selected works of Hildegard E. Peplau* (pp. 205-229). New York: Springer.

Peplau, H. E. (1989c). Loneliness. In A. W. O'Toole & S. R. Welt (Eds.), *Interpersonal theory in nursing practice: Selected works of Hildegard E. Peplau* (pp. 255-269). New York: Springer.

Peplau, H. E. (1989d). Theory: The professional dimension. In A. W. O'Toole & S. R. Welt (Eds.), *Interpersonal theory in nursing practice: Selected works of Hildegard E. Peplau* (pp. 21-41). New York: Springer.

Peplau, H. E. (1989e). Therapeutic nurse-patient interaction. In A. W. O'Toole & S. R. Welt (Eds.), *Interpersonal theory in nursing practice: Selected works of Hildegard E. Peplau* (pp. 192-204). New York: Springer.

Peplau, H. E. (1991/1952). *Interpersonal relations in nursing.* New York: Springer. (reissued)

Saltzman, C., Leutgert, M., Roth, C., Creaser, J., & Howard, L. (1976). Formation of a therapeutic relationship: Experiences during the initial phase as predictors of treatment duration and outcome. *Journal of Consulting and Clinical Psychology, 44,* 546-555.

Sills, G. M. (1978). Hildegard E. Peplau: Leader, practitioner, academician, scholar and theorist. *Perspectives in Psychiatric Care, 16*(3), 122-128.

Smith, D. E. (1990). *Conceptual practices of power.* Toronto: University of Toronto Press.

Sullivan, H. S. (1952). *The interpersonal theory of psychiatry.* New York: Norton.

Thompson, L. (1986). Peplau's theory: An application to short-term individual therapy. *Journal of Psychosocial Nursing, 24*(8), 26-31.

Tudor, G. E. (1952). A sociopsychiatric nursing approach to intervention in a problem of mutual withdrawal on a mental hospital ward. *Psychiatry: Journal for the study of Interpersonal Processes, 15*(2).

Weinert, C. (1987). A social support measure: PRQ85. *Nursing Research, 36,* 273-277.

Bibliography

Beeber, L., Anderson, C. A., & Sills, G. M. (1990). Peplau's theory in practice. *Nursing Science Quarterly, 3*(1), 6-8.

Belcher, J., & Fish, L. (1980). Hildegard E. Peplau. In J. B. George (Ed.), *Nursing theories: The base for professional nursing practice* (pp. 43-60). Englewood Cliffs, NJ: Prentice Hall.

Blake, M. (1980). The Peplau developmental model for nursing practice. In J. P. Riehl & C. Roy (Eds.), *Conceptual models for nursing practice* (2nd ed.) (pp. 53-59) . New York: Appleton-Century-Crofts.

Buchanan, J. (1993). The teacher-student relationship: The heart of nursing education. In M. Rather (Ed.), *Transforming RN education: Dialogue and debate* (pp. 304-323). New York: NLN Publications.

Burd, S. F., & Marshall, M. A. (Eds.). (1971). *Some clinical approaches to psychiatric nursing.* London: Macmillan.

Carey, E. T., Rasmussen, L., Searey, B., & Stark, N. L. (1986). Hildegard E. Peplau: Psychodynamic nursing. In A. Marriner (Ed.), *Nursing theorists and their work* (pp. 181-195). Toronto: C. V. Mosby.

Chinn, P. L., & Jacobs, M. K. (1983). *Theory and nursing: A systematic approach.* Toronto: C. V. Mosby.

Choiniere, J. (1991). *Clients' perceptions of nurse behaviors that facilitate trust in nurse-client relationships.* Unpublished master's thesis, Saint Joseph College, West Hartford, CT.

Field, W. E. (1978). *Psychotherapy of Hildegard Peplau.* New Braunfels, TX: P. S. F. Productions.

Field, W. E., & Ruelke, W. (1973). Hallucinations and how to deal with them. *American Journal of Nursing, 73*(4), 638-640.

Fitzpatrick, J., & Whall, A. (1983). *Conceptual models of nursing: Analysis and application.* Bowie, MD: Robert J. Brady.

56   HILDEGARD E. PEPLAU

Fitzpatrick, J., Whall, A., Johnson, R., & Floyd, J. (1982). *Nursing models and their psychiatric mental health applications*. Bowie, MD: Robert J. Brady.

Forchuk, C. (1990). Peplau's interpersonal theory. In A. Baumann, N. Johnson, & D. Atai-Otaong (Eds.), *Decision making in psychiatric and psychosocial nursing* (pp. 22-23). Toronto: B. C. Decker.

Forchuk, C. (1991). A comparison of the works of Peplau and Orlando. *Archives of Psychiatric Nursing, 5*(1), 38-45.

Forchuk, C. (1991). Conceptualizing the environment of the individual with a chronic mental illness. *Issues in Mental Health Nursing, 12,* 159-170.

Forchuk, C. (1991). Peplau's theory: Concepts and their relations. *Nursing Science Quarterly, 4*(2), 54-60.

Forchuk, C. (1992). The orientation phase of the nurse-client relationship: Testing Peplau's theory. Unpublished doctoral dissertation, Wayne State University, Detroit, MI.

Forchuk, C. (1992). The orientation phase: How long does it take? *Perspectives in Psychiatric Care, 28*(4), 7-10.

Forchuk, C., Beaton, S., Crawford, L., Ide, L., Voorberg, N., & Bethune, J. (1989). Incorporating Peplau's theory and case management. *Journal of Psychosocial Nursing, 27*(2), 35-38.

Forchuk, C., & Brown, B. (1989). Establishing a nurse-client relationship. *Journal of Psychosocial Nursing, 27*(2), 30-34.

Forchuk, C., & Voorberg, N. (1991). Evaluating a community mental health program. *Canadian Journal of Nursing Administration, 4*(6) 16-20.

Gehrs, M. (1991). *The relationship between the working alliance and rehabilitation outcomes of clients with schizophrenia.* Unpublished master's thesis, University of Toronto, Ontario, Canada.

Goering, P. N., & Stylianos, S. K. (1988). Exploring the helping relationship between schizophrenic client and rehabilitation therapist. *American Journal of Orthopsychiatry, 58*(2), 271-280.

Gregg, D. (1954). The psychiatric nurse's role. *American Journal of Nursing, 54*(7), 848-851. (reprinted In D. Mereness, work cited, Vol. 1, pp. 178-185.)

Gregg, D. (1978). Hildegard E. Peplau: Her contributions. *Perspectives in Psychiatric Care, 16*(3), 118-121.

Hays, J. (1966). Analysis of nurse-patient communication. *Nursing Outlook, 14*(9), 32-35.

Hays, J., & Larson, K. (1963). *Interacting with patients.* New York: Macmillan.

Hays, J., & Myers, J. (1964). Learning in the nurse-patient relationship. *Perspectives in Psychiatric Care, 2,* 20.

Hirschmann, M. J. (1989). Psychiatric and mental health nurses' beliefs about therapeutic paradox. *Journal of Child Psychiatric Nursing, 2*(1), 7-13.

Lego, S. (1980). The one-to-one nurse-patient relationship. *Perspectives in Psychiatric Care, 18,* 67-89.

Lemmer, B. (1988). Care plan for a man receiving domiciliary care, using Peplau's model of nursing. In B. Collister (Ed.), *Psychiatric nursing: Person to person.* London: Edward Arnold.

Manaser, J. C., & Werner, A. M. (1964). *Instruments for the study of nurse-patient interaction.* New York: Macmillan.

Martin, M. L., Forchuk, C., Santopinto, M., & Butcher, H. (1992). Alternative approaches to nursing practice: Application of Peplau, Rogers, and Parse. *Nursing Science Quarterly, 5*(8), 80-85.

O'Toole, A. W., & Welt, S. R. (Eds.). (1989). *Interpersonal theory in nursing practice: Selected works of Hildegard E. Peplau.* New York: Springer.

Parse, R. R. (1987). *Nursing science: Major paradigms, theories, and critiques.* Toronto: W. B. Saunders.

Peplau, H. E. (1952). *Interpersonal relations in nursing.* New York: G. P. Putnam.

Peplau, H. E. (l952). Psychiatric nurses family groups. *American Journal of Nursing, 52,* 1475-1477.

Peplau, H. E. (1960, May). Anxiety in the mother-infant relationship. *Nurses Weekly,* 134.

Peplau, H. E. (1960). Talking with patients. *American Journal of Nursing, 60,* 964+.

Peplau, H. E. (1962). Interpersonal techniques: The crux of psychiatric nursing. *American Journal of Nursing, 62,* 50-54.

Peplau, H. E. (1964). *Basic principals of patient counselling,* Philadelphia: Smith, Kline and French Laboratories.

Peplau, H. E. (1965). The heart of nursing: Interpersonal relations. *Canadian Nurse, 61,* 273.

Peplau, H. E. (1967). Interpersonal relations and the work of the industrial nurse. *American Association of Industrial Nurses Journal, 15*(11), 7-12.

Peplau, H. E. (1969). Professional closeness - as a special kind of involvement with a patient, client, or family group. *Nursing Forum, 8*(4), 342-360.

Peplau, H. E. (1971). Anxiety. In S. F. Burd & M. A. Marshall (Eds.), *Some clinical approaches to psychiatric nursing* (pp. 323-327). London: MacMillan.

Peplau, H. E. (1971). Process and concept of learning. In S. F. Burd & M. A. Marshall (Eds.), *Some clinical approaches to psychiatric nursing* (pp. 333-336). London: Macmillan.

Peplau, H. E. (Speaker). (1973). *Anxiety* (audio tape). San Antonio, TX: P. S. F. Productions.

Peplau, H. E. (Speaker). (1973). *The concept of psychotherapy* (audio tape). San Antonio, TX: P. S. F. Productions.

Peplau, H. E. (Speaker). (1973). *Illness maintaining systems.* (audio tape) San Antonio, TX: P. S. F. Productions.

Peplau, H. E. (Speaker). (1973). *Language and its relation to thought disorders.* (audio tape) San Antonio, TX: P. S. F. Productions.

Peplau, H. E. (Speaker). (1973). *The orientation phase* (audio tape). San Antonio, TX: P. S. F. Productions.

Peplau, H. E. (Speaker). (1973). *The resolution phase* (audio tape). San Antonio, TX: P. S. F. Productions.

Peplau, H. E. (Speaker). (1973). *The working phase* (audio tape). San Antonio, TX: P. S. F. Productions.

Peplau, H. E. (1976). What future for nursing? *American Operating Room Nursing Journal, 24,* 217-235.

Peplau, H. E. (1977). The changing view of nursing. *International Nursing Review, 24*(2), 43-45.

Peplau, H. E. (1987). Interpersonal constructs for nursing practice. *Nurse Education Today, 7*(5), 201-208.

58 HILDEGARD E. PEPLAU

Peplau, H. E. (1987). Nursing science: A historical perspective. In R. Parse (Ed.), *Nursing science: Major paradigms, theories, and critiques* (pp. 13-30). Toronto: W. B. Saunders.

Peplau, H. E. (1988). The art and science of nursing: Similarities, differences and relations. *Nursing Science Quarterly, 1,* 8-15.

Peplau, H. E. (1988/1952). *Interpersonal relations in nursing.* London: Macmillan. (reissued)

Peplau, H. E. (1989). Anxiety, self and hallucinations. In A. W. O'Toole & S. R. Welt (Eds.), *Interpersonal theory in nursing practice: Selected works of Hildegard E. Peplau* (pp. 270-326). New York: Springer.

Peplau, H. E. (1989). Investigative counseling. In A. W. O'Toole & S. R. Welt (Eds.), *Interpersonal theory in nursing practice: Selected works of Hildegard E. Peplau* (pp. 205-229). New York: Springer.

Peplau, H. E. (1989). Loneliness. In A. W. O'Toole & S. R. Welt (Eds.), *Interpersonal theory in nursing practice: Selected works of Hildegard E. Peplau* (pp. 255-269). New York: Springer.

Peplau, H. E. (1989). Theory: The professional dimension. In A. W. O'Toole & S. R. Welt (Eds.), *Interpersonal theory in nursing practice: Selected works of Hildegard E. Peplau* (pp. 21-41). New York: Springer.

Peplau, H. E. (1989). Therapeutic nurse-patient interaction. In A. W. O'Toole & S. R. Welt (Eds.), *Interpersonal theory in nursing practice: Selected works of Hildegard E. Peplau* (pp. 192-204). New York: Springer.

Peplau, H. E. (1991/1952). *Interpersonal relations in nursing.* New York: Springer. (reissued)

Rix, G. (1988). Care plan for an aggressive person, based on Peplau's model of nursing. In B. Collister (Ed.), *Psychiatric nursing: Person to person* (pp. 119-127). London: Edward Arnold.

Sills, G. M. (1978). Hildegard E. Peplau: Leader, practitioner, academician, scholar and theorist. *Perspectives in Psychiatric Care, 16*(3), 122-128.

Silva, M. C. (1986). Research testing nursing theory: State of the art. *Advances in Nursing Science, 9*(1), 1-11.

Smith, M. J. (1988). Perspectives on nursing science. *Nursing Science Quarterly, 1,* 80-85.

Sullivan, H. S. (1952). *The interpersonal theory of psychiatry.* New York: Norton.

Thompson, L. (1986). Peplau's theory: An application to short-term individual therapy. *Journal of Psychosocial Nursing, 24*(8), 26-31.

Tudor, G. E. (1952). A sociopsychiatric nursing approach to intervention in a problem of mutual withdrawal on a mental hospital ward. *Psychiatry: Journal for the study of Interpersonal Processes, 15*(2).

Walker, L. O., & Avant, K. C. (1988). *Strategies for theory construction in nursing* (2nd ed.). Norwalk, CT: Appleton & Lange.

Woolridge, P. J., Schmitt, M. H., Skipper, J. K., & Leonard, R. C. (1983). *Behavioral science and nursing theory.* Toronto: C. V. Mosby.

About the Author

Cheryl Forchuk, R.N., Ph.D., is a Clinical Nurse Specialist at Hamilton Psychiatric Hospital, an Associate Clinical Professor at McMaster University, Hamilton, Ontario, Canada, and has a private practice in stress management. She received her B.Sc. in Nursing and B.A. in psychology from the University of Windsor. She received her M.Sc. in Nursing with a clinical specialty in mental health nursing from the University of Toronto and her Ph.D. from the College of Nursing at Wayne State University in Detroit, Michigan. Dr. Forchuk has published on many topics including: denial, health promotion, sexuality, and Peplau's interpersonal theory of nursing. Her current research includes exploring the orientation phase of the nurse-client relationship.